Lose Weight:
On a Healthy
Vegetarian Diet

I0423722

CHARLES BENSON

Table of Contents

Chapter 1- An Overview of Weight Loss and A Vegetarian Diet 3

Chapter 2- Vegetarian Diets for Weight Loss................15

Chapter 3- Vegetarian Diet Planner 29

Chapter 4- Recipes for a Vegetarian Diet......................35

Chapter 5- Tips to Maximize the Use of Vegetarian Diets for Weight Loss 76

Conclusion...83

Chapter 1- An Overview of Weight Loss and A Vegetarian Diet

If you are thinking about losing weight, you know that it is not only about dropping a pants size or two. There is more to losing weight than looking better in your clothes, in fact, losing weight can be very beneficial to your health as well.

Of course, weight loss will make you look better, you will have more energy and you will feel better about yourself, but the health benefits are going to ensure you live longer and have a higher quality of life.

Being overweight increases your risk of many diseases and by losing weight, you can reduce your risk of these diseases. Diseases such as heart disease, diabetes, high blood pressure, sleep apnea and even some cancers are more prevalent in those that are overweight. Many of these diseases can be completely eliminated simply by losing weight and changing what you are putting into your body.

On top of reducing your risks for disease or even reversing diseases that you are already suffering from, losing weight is going to help you feel more energetic. If you have been feeling sluggish, exhausted or just think that you could be getting more done each day, losing weight will help you to get the energy you are looking for.

Many people feel as if they are in complete control of their lives, they run businesses, take care of everything that they need to handle every day and yet they do not feel as if they are able to take control of their weight. By using a vegetarian diet, you can finally get control of your weight, thus finally taking control of your life.

Studies have shown that even though it is extremely unfair, those that are overweight are often thought of as lazy or less educated than those that are thinner. Those of the opposite sex are naturally more attracted to those that are healthy and not overweight, and you have a higher chance of getting the job that you want if you are a healthy weight.

All of these are benefits of losing weight, but what are the risks of remaining overweight? Those that are overweight increase their risk of high blood pressure, high cholesterol, type 2 diabetes, heart disease, stroke, gallbladder disease, osteoarthritis, sleep apnea, asthma and other breathing issues, cancer, mental illness and pain in the body.

Those that are overweight, are at a higher risk of being depressed and suffering from anxiety while those that are of normal weight tend to be able to relax and are less stressed than those that are overweight.

A Look at The Stats

When most people are focusing on losing weight, the most important numbers to them are the ones that are on the scale as well as the total number of calories they are eating and how many minutes they are working out.

There are, however, other numbers that we need to look at when it comes to weight loss. The first number is 2. This is the percentage of people that are successful when they are trying to lose weight using a diet. This means that only 2 percent of people that try various diets are actually successful at losing the weight and keeping it off.

You see, most diets are restrictive, they force you to count calories and deprive yourself of the food that your body craves. Diets simply do not work, and this number is proof of that. The good news is, that what you are going to learn throughout this book is not a diet, but a lifestyle, one that will guarantee your weight loss success.

The next number is 20 billion. This is the amount of money that is made each year in the US alone by the weight loss industry. This includes weight loss surgeries, diet plans, and diet pills.

108 million is the number of people that are on a diet at any given time in the United States. Each of

these 108 million people will try to diet on average of five times before giving up and not being successful.

85 percent is the number of people that are purchasing weight loss products that are female. This shows us that women are very concerned about their weight and that they are struggling to lose weight and keep it off.

220,000 is the number of people in the US that go through weight loss surgery in an average year.

2 million dollars is the average amount that celebrities get paid to endorse a weight loss program or product. Think about that the next time that you see a celebrity endorsing a product. For 2 million dollars, I bet you would endorse any product, whether you thought it worked or not.

33,000 dollars is the average amount per pound lost that each celebrity is paid when endorsing a product. Now if that is not motivation to get out and exercise, I don't know what is.

1 in 5. This is the number of deaths that are caused by weight-related issues.

According to the Center for Disease Control, 1 in 3 Americans suffer from obesity. Non-Hispanic blacks are reported to have the highest rate of obesity, according to the CDC, almost 48 percent are considered obese. This is followed closely by Hispanics at almost 43 percent, whites, at 33 percent, and Asians at 11 percent.

The obesity rate for those 40-59 is higher than other age groups, almost 40 percent being considered obese. 40 percent of those 20-39 are considered obese, and 35 percent of those that are over 60 are considered obese.

Finally, according to the CDC, women that have lower incomes and are less educated are more likely to be overweight than women with higher incomes and are more educated.

Types of Diets that are Out There

There are many different diet programs out there, some of them people have seen success with while others have not been successful at all. I want to start with the three-hour diet, when you are on this diet, you will eat every three hours. Your meals will be very small, and although there are no restrictions on what you can eat, the portion sizes are highly restricted. The idea is that by eating every three hours, you will keep your metabolic rate high thus causing you to lose weight.

The Atkins diet focuses on eating a lot of protein as well as low starch vegetables while cutting out the simple carb ensuring that the blood sugar does not spike. The idea is that by reducing the amount of simple carbs you are eating; you will naturally reduce the amount of weight you are carrying around. There are however many problems with this diet and studies have shown that it can cause heart disease to worsen.

The Best Life Diet is a program that tries to focus on the reason you are overeating and encourages you to change the way you are eating and exercising by changing your emotional state. It claims that by focusing on the reason you are overeating and not exercising, and dealing with that issue, you will begin eating healthy and exercising regularly. The problem that I find with this diet is that many people overeat because they are feeling depressed, they are depressed because they are overweight, and they are not going to feel better until they begin losing weight. Each of these issues has to be dealt with separately but simultaneously as well. Simply treating a person's emotional issues is not going to cause them to lose weight.

There is also a diet called the Blood Type Diet. This diet claims that you should eat certain foods depending on your blood type and that there are certain foods you should avoid according to your blood type. The truth is, our bodies, no matter what our blood type, have to have certain foods, and certain nutrients. It does not matter what your blood type is, if you cut any of these foods out of your diet, your body is not going to function properly.

Of course, there are many other diets, the cabbage soup diet, the caveman diet, the fat flush diet, the French Women Don't Get Fat diet, the Glycemic Index diet, the Grapefruit diet, the Hormone diet, Jenny Craig, Macrobiotic Diet, the Master Cleanse

Diet, the Mediterranean diet, the New Beverly Hills diet, Nutrisystem, the South Beach diet, Weight Watchers, and the Zone diet.

These are just a few of the diets that are available, and if you take a look at the list, it is no wonder that so many people are struggling to lose weight. Each of these diets claims that they will help you lose weight quickly and keep it off, but if this were true, wouldn't everyone we know be thin, fit and healthy?

Vegetarian Diet to Lose Weight Vs. Other Diets

Now that you have learned a bit about the other diet programs out there, you may be thinking that a vegetarian diet is just another fad diet that claims to help you lose weight. I want to prove to you that a vegetarian diet will help you not only lose weight but that it will help you become a happier, healthier person as well.

Studies have shown that when the consumption of meats such as red meat, chicken, fish, and pork are limited, it results in improved moods. This is because there is a specific amino acid in meat that causes mood disturbances.

A vegetarian diet can also help to reduce the symptoms of psoriasis, reduce the symptoms of diabetes, reverse heart disease, reduce the risk of developing cataracts, lower cholesterol, reduce the risk of stroke, kidney stones, reduce weight and improve nutrition.

When it comes to comparing a vegetarian diet to other diets, on the market, the main benefit that makes a vegetarian diet stand out from the rest is that it is healthy. Most diets are restrictive, they do not allow you to eat the foods that your body needs and many of them depend on processed prepackaged foods or pills. These diets are unsuccessful because of this.

However, when you eat a vegetarian diet, you are eliminating the processed foods. You are giving your body the nutrients that it needs to ensure that it is functioning properly, and you never have to worry about feeling hungry.

Most diets are just that; they are diets that are used temporarily as an attempt to lose weight quickly. A vegetarian diet, however, is one that will be eaten for the rest of your life. You don't have to worry about just getting through this diet because you know that for the rest of your life, you are going to eat healthy, vegetarian meals.

According to one study done by the University of South Carolina, a vegetarian diet will help you to lose about 7.9 percent more body weight than those diets that contain meat. This means that while a person that eats meat may lose five pounds, a person that is on a vegetarian diet will lose about 8 pounds. While the person that lost the five pounds may be losing weight on their diet, chances are they are going to gain it back because remember, only 2 percent of those that lose weight on diets, keep the weight off.

Those that lose with a vegetarian diet are more likely to keep the weight off, as long as they stick to the lifestyle change and do not go back to filling their bodies with junk after they lose the weight.

The great thing about a vegetarian diet is that you do not have to worry about counting calories or going hungry. The idea of a vegetarian diet is to allow you to feel full while getting the nutrients that your body needs. This may seem a bit extreme for some people, but for others, it is very liberating, not having to count calories and worry about getting the nutrition that you need while still being able to lose weight, improve your health and your happiness may be just what you need.

Chapter 2- Vegetarian Diets for Weight Loss

Counting calories can be a thing of the past. Many studies have shown that the real way to lose weight, keep it off and maintain a healthy body is to eat a vegetarian diet.

We have already talked about some of the benefits of a vegetarian diet as it pertains to improving health and I want to talk a bit more about the benefits, but first, I want to spend some time talking about what a vegetarian diet really is.

Some people consider themselves vegetarian, but they are really eating very few vegetables. You need to realize that just because you live on potato chips and soda does not make you a vegetarian. It makes you a very unhealthy person.

A vegetarian diet will not include any meat, meaning a vegetarian will not eat pork, beef, chicken, veal, fish, or any other type of meat. A vegan, on the other hand, will not eat any animal product, meaning they will not drink milk, eat cheese or anything that has been made with animal products.

Some vegetarians do eat eggs, while others remove the eggs from their diet as well. It all depends on what type of vegetarian you would like to be.

A vegetarian diet can be healthier than other diets if you make sure you are eating the healthy foods that you need instead of the junk that you do not need. For example, instead of eating a bag of chips for lunch, you will need to make sure you are eating a healthy meal full of fruits, veggies, nuts, grains or beans.

Each meal needs to be balanced, and you need to ensure that you are not chasing it by a bunch of fizzy soda. Of course soda is a vegetarian drink, but it is packed full of calories, and there is no nutritional value in soda, so although it is technically vegetarian, it will still blow your diet. A true vegetarian diet is going to be one that is made up of mostly plants.

The challenges you will face.

When you choose to start eating a vegetarian diet, you are going to face a few challenges. The first one is usually other people. When I first became a vegetarian, it seemed as if everyone I knew wanted to fight me on the choice. I had people telling me that I was going to get sick, that because I suffered from anemia, I was not going to be able to stick to a vegetarian diet, and that eating a vegetarian diet would affect my looks, causing me to look drained, pale and sickly.

At first, this can be overwhelming, and it can make you begin to question your decision of becoming a vegetarian, but it does not have to if you have the right information.

The first thing that you need to know about is malnutrition. When we think about malnutrition, we often think about those that are super thin, their bellies swollen and their face, sunken in. We think of those that are starving. But, in the US, that is not the face of malnutrition, in fact, those that are lacking nutrition in their diets are often the overweight.

The reason for this is because most of the food that they are eating is processed, it is food that was created in a lab and not grown from the ground. Therefore, they are not getting the vitamins and minerals that they need which is what truly leads to malnutrition.

You see, while these people are eating enough calories, generally more than they really need, they are doing their bodies no good because the food that they are eating does not contain the vitamins and minerals that their body needs to function properly.

Imagine what happens when your body is hungry and even though you fill it, you do not give it what it really needs. The body is going to continue to crave what it needs, which is one of the reasons we have a generation of people that never seem to understand what it is to feel full.

Studies have shown that about 85 percent of people in the United States are suffering from malnutrition. I have told you all of this so that when someone comes at you, telling you that what you are eating is going to be detrimental to your health, you will be able to remind yourself, that you do not want to be part of the 85 percent of overweight people that are malnourished.

Of course, just like everyone struggles to fill the gaps in their diet, you will have some issues if you are eating a vegetarian diet, but careful planning is going to ensure that you are getting all of the vitamins and nutrients that you need.

Another challenge that I faced was a lack of variety. There are only so many ways that you can cook the same vegetables, and although we do have some variety in what is available where I am from, most of the foods we eat are seasonal.

This means that you will need to plan ahead when it comes to your meals and that you might have to learn how to cook differently than you have before. The reason is because if you have a limited variety of vegetables and fruits, you can become bored quickly and start looking for different flavors.

One of the ways that you can add variety to your diet is to look each week for one new vegetable to add to your meal plan. Try new vegetables and fruits that you have never considered trying before and work those into your weekly meal plan.

You may have to turn to frozen fruits and vegetables to get some extra variety in your diet, especially in the winter months when fresh fruits and vegetables are not in season.

Now that you know what a vegetarian diet is and a few facts about how the diet is healthier for you than it is diets that contain meat, I want to go over a few more benefits of the vegetarian diet.

Studies have shown that eating a vegetarian diet reduces the risk of obesity. You are going to be eating reduced saturated fats, which means that your cardiovascular health is going to improve greatly.

You are going to also ensure that you are getting enough of the right carbohydrates. Carbohydrates are what provides the body with energy. Many people eat a large amount of simple carbohydrates, such as breads, pastas and baked goods. These simple carbohydrates will work like coffee, giving you a quick energy boost but because there is so much energy and it is impossible for you to burn it off, the extra energy will be stored as fat.

When you eat complex carbohydrates, they digest slower, which means that they release the energy in the body which means that you will have sustained energy throughout the entire day.

You will be eating a high fiber diet which means that you are going to have a very healthy digestive system.

On top of all of this, your body is going to be able to heal itself when you provide it with the nutrients that it needs. You can heal allergies, asthma, behavior disorders, mental disorders, and many other diseases.

Food Composition and Functions

When it comes to eating a vegetarian diet, you are going to be filling your body with lots of healthy vitamins and nutrients. Of course, you know that these nutrients are good for you, but you may be wondering exactly what it is that you are putting into your body and what is the reason for eating these specific nutrients.

I want to cover just a few of the vitamins and minerals that you are going to find in your fruits and vegetables as well as what the function of these vitamins and minerals are in the body.

We have talked a bit about complex carbohydrates, but it is important for you to understand that complex carbohydrates do not make you fat. Overeating and not getting enough exercise is what makes you fat, complex carbohydrates are necessary for your body to function properly.

Complex carbohydrates are used by the body as a source of energy. As I stated earlier, complex carbohydrates are going to give your body the energy it needs over a long period of time instead of in short bursts.

When you are trying to lose weight, you will need to eat several servings of complex carbohydrates every day, but you need to stop consuming them about 4 hours before you go to bed, otherwise, your body cannot turn them into energy, and they will instead be turned to fat.

Complex carbohydrates include, but are not limited to: Legumes, sweet potatoes, whole grain bread, whole grain pasta, oats, brown rice, quinoa, fruit, whole grains and beans.

If you do not eat enough complex carbohydrates, your energy levels will drop, and you will not be able to get through your day or through your workout.

Vitamin C is the next thing that I want to talk about. We all know that vitamin C is important for us to have healthy immune systems, and it supports healthy immune system function. What you probably did not know was that vitamin C is also crucial for the health of your teeth and gums, it works to ensure you do not have allergies, works as an antioxidant, plays a vital role in iron absorption, fights against vision loss, plays a role in the healing of wounds and even contributes to the regeneration of skin and collagen.

Did you know that thiamine was one of the first recognized vitamins and is vital to the function of the entire body? You must have thiamine in order to have a healthy nervous system and to ensure proper muscle function. It plays a role in digestion, muscle cell repair and you cannot metabolize carbohydrates without thiamine. Thiamine is also known as Vitamin B1. All B vitamins play a huge role in the amount of energy that you have as well as the way your entire body functions and it is important for you to ensure you are getting enough of them all.

Riboflavin is the next vitamin that I want to talk about. Riboflavin is another B vitamin, B2 to be more specific, and it is vital for the growth of the body as well as the production of red blood cells.

Niacin is also known as Vitamin B3. The function of Niacin is to turn food into glucose, which is later turned into energy.

Vitamin A is important for you to maintain healthy teeth, skin, and eyes. It is also vital for the skeletal system as well as your soft tissue.

Finally, proteins are vital for the function of every cell of the body. Each cell is made up of proteins, and proteins are needed to repair the cells, especially as our bodies grow. Proteins are also used for energy. This means that if you take in more protein than your body needs for maintenance and repairs, your body will use the protein for energy. However, if your body does not need the energy, it will just like carbohydrates, be turned to fat. Protein is also a must when it comes to balancing and producing hormones in the body.

Foods That are on a Basic Vegetarian Diet

Not eating meat or changing to a vegetarian diet does not mean that you have to eat bland foods or that you cannot take pleasure in cooking your foods. However, you do want to avoid the highly processed foods that are meant to take the place of meat. These types of food may be fine if you are just starting when it comes to getting the meat out of your diet, but they are not healthy foods and they are not going to help you lose the weight that you are looking to lose. Here are some of the foods that you want to begin incorporating into your vegetarian diet:

Dairy: Soy milk, Almond milk, Coconut milk, Rice milk or Hemp milk, dairy free cheese, dairy free sour cream and soy yogurt.

Protein: Beans, seeds, chickpeas, hummus, tofu, and nuts.

Grains: Quinoa, oats, couscous, brown rice, and whole wheat pastas, breads and tortillas.

Vegetables: Tomatoes, carrots, lettuce, spinach, Kale, artichoke, beetroot, asparagus, bell pepper, Brussel sprout, broccoli, cabbage, celery, cauliflower, corn, cucumbers, corn, green beans, eggplant, mushrooms, cauliflower, fennel, chives, leeks, avocado, peas, sweet potato, pumpkin, onions, radish, zucchini, squash and so on.

Fruits: Melons, strawberries, blueberries, raspberries, apples, grapes, cherries, cranberries, oranges, pomegranate, grapefruit, lemons, limes, kiwi, bananas, dates, nectarine, plums, fig, raisins, mango, peach and so on.

You will also use vegetable broth and bouillon when cooking instead of beef or chicken.

You will also use flax seeds, Chia seeds, when cooking and baking.

How many Calories Should You Eat?

The first thing that you need to know when it comes to the amount of calories that you will be eating a vegetarian diet is that you should never eat less than 1200 calories per day even if you are on a diet. However, most women are going to need about 2,000 calories per day, and most men are going to need about 2500.

You really do not have to worry about counting calories when you are on a vegetarian diet as long as you are not snacking on potato chips, chocolate and other highly processed junk foods that are providing your body with no nutritional value.

For a woman that needs 2,000 calories per day, she should aim for 3, 500 calorie meals and 2, 250 calorie snacks.

For a woman that needs 1200 calories per day, she would aim for 3, 300 calorie meals and 2, 150 calorie snacks.

For a man that needs 2500, calories per day, he should aim for 3, 625 calorie meals and 2, 313 calorie snacks.

For a man that needs 1700 calories per day, he should aim for 3, 425 calorie meals and 2, 213 calorie snacks.

Your caloric need per day is going to depend on the amount of weight you want to lose per week and your activity level. You see, you have to have 3,500 calories less per week than you do right now in order to lose 1 pound per week. Therefore, if you want to lose 2 pounds per week, you will need a deficit of 7,000 calories each week.

This comes not only from the food that you are eating but the amount of calories you are burning as you exercise as well. So if you are a 200 pound woman, eating 2300 calories per day, you will want to cut your caloric intake back to about 1200 calories. This gives you a 1100 calorie deficit each day or 7,700 per week, meaning that you are going to lose 2 pounds per week.

Now let's say you exercise 30 minutes each morning and burn 300 calories, this means that you can now eat 1500 calories per day and still lose the same 2 pounds per week.

Chapter 3- Vegetarian Diet Planner

Before we get into talking about your weekly diet plan, I want to make it very clear that you simply cannot eat as much as you want when it comes to a vegetarian diet. All of the vegetarian foods have calories, calories, if not burned up as energy that will turn to fat.

This means that you do need to pay attention to the amount of food that you are eating on a regular basis. You see, even though you may be able to sit down and polish off an entire salad meant for a family, blend 4 bananas into a low-fat ice cream for desert and then still have enough room for several oranges as a snack, eating this amount of food is going to do nothing more than make you fat.

Yes, you may see some weight loss, but what you are going to find is that even though you are losing weight, your body fat for your weight is going to be very very high which means you are going to be very unhealthy.

When you are eating, especially when you are on a diet, you do want to give your body the food that it needs when you are hungry, and I will be the first to tell you that on this diet, you are going to be hungry when it is meal time and snack time. However, you need to realize that after you have eaten your meal or snack, although your body feels as if you could eat more, there is no need for it, and you do not need to go back for seconds or thirds. Doing so will only defeat your purpose.

We need to remind ourselves that we are not to stop eating because our stomach is full. Of course, there are special occasions that we stuff ourselves to the point of exploding such as Thanksgiving, but that type of behavior does not happen every day.

Instead, we need to realize, we are no longer hungry, walk away from the kitchen and move on to our next activity. The point in all of this is that just like if you were eating any other foods, you can get fat if you overeat on a vegetarian diet, you will simply be a well-nourished fat person instead of a malnourished one.

I have already told you in this book that unless you have a well thought out plan, you will struggle with a vegetarian diet and chances are that you will not see the success that you are looking for. For that reason, in this chapter, I want to give you a seven-day meal plan that will ensure you are able to see the success you so desire. In the next chapter, I will go over the recipes with you.

Day 1-

Breakfast- Green Apple Oats

Lunch- Veggie Humus Wrap

Dinner-Baked Ziti

Day 2-

Breakfast- Smashed Avocado Toast With Veggies

Lunch-Lentil Soup

Dinner- Eggplant sandwiches

Day 3-

Breakfast- Breakfast Veggie Tacos

Lunch-Vegetarian Chili

Dinner-Zucchini Grinders

Day 4-

Breakfast- Veggie Bagel Sandwich

Lunch- Pasta Salad

Dinner-Black bean veggie burgers

Day 5-

Breakfast- Breakfast Burritos

Lunch- Lentil and Chickpea Salad

Dinner- Quinoa and black beans

Day 6-

Breakfast- Green Smoothie

Lunch-Kale and Apple Salad

Dinner- Veggie Pizza

Day 7-

Breakfast- Fruit Salad

Lunch- Miso Soup

Dinner- Spinach Enchiladas

You can also add in snacks in between your meals, fruit, veggies with hummus dip, and smoothies are all great snacks for vegetarians.

Chapter 4- Recipes for a Vegetarian Diet

In the last chapter, we went over a full week of meals for a vegetarian diet. I have done this to give you not only an idea of the types of meals that you can eat on a vegetarian diet but also to help you get started in your new lifestyle.

Eating vegetarian does not have to be boring, and I hope that you have come to know that by the meal plan I laid out for you, but a meal plan will do you no good if you don't know how to cook the meals. Therefore, in this chapter, I want to cover how to cook each of the recipes in the previous chapter. Remember, nothing has to be bland, and you can enjoy cooking even though you are eating a vegetarian diet.

Breakfasts

Green Apple Oats:

You will need- 1 cup of steel cut or rolled oats, 2 cups of water or almond milk (almond milk will add more to the total calories per serving), 1 green apple.

Begin by dicing the green apple. Then mix your oats with your water or almond milk, bringing it to a boil. Allow this to simmer for a few minutes. This will make creamy oatmeal, however, if you like your oatmeal a little less creamy, place the milk or water in your pan first, bringing it to a boil then stir in your oats.

You can wait to add the apple until the oats are cooked or add it in while they are cooking, it is up to you. Allow the oats to cook on low for about 15 minutes, stirring them occasionally, ensuring that they do not burn to the bottom of the pain.

Smashed Avocado Toast With Veggies-

You will need:

2 slices of Ezekiel bread

2 eggs, fried in coconut oil

1 avocado

½ of a purple onion that has been sliced thinly

½ a cup of your choice bell pepper, sliced thinly

4 asparagus spears that have been sliced in half

1 tablespoon of coconut oil

The juice from ½ of a lime

Salt and pepper to taste

Begin by melting the coconut oil in a skillet over medium heat. After the oil has melted, place the purple onion slices, pepper slices, asparagus, salt and pepper in the skillet sautéing for about five minutes. Squeeze the juice from one half of a lime over the vegetable mixture and allow to cook for about two more minutes.

While this is cooking, place bread in a toaster, when it is finished toasting, smash avocado on the toast, followed by the vegetables then the fried egg. Serve.

Breakfast Veggie Tacos-

You will need:

For the veggie filling:

2 teaspoons of coconut oil

1 white onion, small, diced

3 cloves of garlic, minced

1 zucchini, sliced lengthwise then cut into 2 inch pieces

1 yellow squash, sliced lengthwise then cut into 2 inch pieces

1 red pepper, removed the seeds and chop

The juice of ½ a lime

Salt, red pepper flakes

For the scrambled eggs, you will need:

6 eggs (already scrambled)

Our choice of hot sauce

Salt and pepper

1 tomato, chopped

You will also need 6 tortillas, whole grain

Garnish with jalapeno, crumbled Feta, and cilantro if desired.

Directions:

You will begin by heating the 2 teaspoons of coconut oil in a skillet over medium heat. Once the oil has melted, you will add onions and a small dash of salt, allowing to cook about five minutes until the onions have become translucent. Next, add in the garlic with a pinch of red pepper flakes and stir. Allow this to cook for about 30 seconds before adding the zucchini, bell pepper, and the yellow squash.

Allow this to cook, until the zucchini and yellow squash have softened. This will take about 7 minutes. Be sure to not overcook because the squash will become squishy.

Remove the pan from the stove before squeezing the lime juice over the mixture then add salt.

Next, you will scramble the eggs in a bowl with a bit of hot sauce, black pepper and salt. Cook the scrambled eggs as desired. When the eggs begin to set, add the chopped tomato, folding it into the scrambled eggs. Once the eggs are done, transfer the mixture into a bowl.

Warm your tortilla shells in a pan, in the oven or in the microwave, filling them with eggs, then veggies and lastly garnishes before serving.

Veggie Bagel Sandwich-

You will need:

1 tablespoon coconut oil

½ an onion, sliced thinly

1 zucchini, sliced thinly lengthwise

1 yellow squash, sliced thinly

1 garlic clove, minced

1 tomato, sliced

Salt and pepper

2 bagels

Unsalted butter

Cream cheese if desired

Directions:

Begin by heating the coconut oil in a skillet over medium heat. Once the coconut oil has melted, add the sliced onions and allow to cook for about 10 minutes or until they begin to turn brown.

Once the onions have begun to turn brown, add in the yellow squash slices and zucchini allowing to cook for about 5 minutes or until they begin to soften and turn brown. Next, you will add in the minced garlic, allowing the mixture to cook for 1 minute.

Next, you will add in the tomatoes, cooking for no more than 2 minutes, ensuring that the tomatoes do not break apart or become overcooked. Add salt and pepper to taste, then remove from heat.

Now you will toast your bagels to light brown, lightly smearing real butter or cream cheese, or both before topping with the veggie mixture. If you do not want to use butter or cream cheese, you do not have to. Serve.

Breakfast Burritos-

You will need:

4 white mushrooms, sliced

2 garlic cloves

¼ a cup of diced red onions

½ of a red pepper, seeded and diced

1 pack of extra firm tofu, crumbled

½ teaspoon cumin,

½ teaspoon chili powder,

½ teaspoon salt

½ teaspoon pepper

½ teaspoon garlic powder

½ teaspoon turmeric

3 teaspoons of water

Wraps

Lime juice

Refried beans,

Salsa

Romaine lettuce

1 avocado, sliced

Cilantro

Directions:

Begin by placing the 3 teaspoons of water in a small bowl. Then add in the chili powder, garlic powder, cumin, salt, turmeric, and pepper. Mix well.

Next, you will place a skillet on the stove, over medium heat, adding in the mushrooms, red pepper, garlic, and onions, allowing to cook for about 7 minutes or until they have started to become soft. You can add in a bit of extra water if you need to.

Now you will crumble the tofu into the pan and top with the spices you mixed in the water. Mix well and allow to cook until the tofu is heated.

While the tofu is cooking you can heat up your refried beans if desired, you can use them cold as well.

Remove the tofu and vegetable mix from the heat and set to the side while you prepare the wraps.

On each wrap, you will place refried beans, lettuce, avocado, salsa, cilantro and top it off with the tofu scramble. Finally, give the burrito a spritz of lime juice and serve.

Green Smoothie-

You will need:

1 cup of fresh kale

1 apple, cored and chopped

1 cucumber, chopped

1 tbsp lemon juice

1 tsp ginger

½ tbsp. Coconut oil

½ tbsp. Maple syrup

5 ice cubes

Protein powder if desired

Begin by placing the kale, apple, cucumber, lemon juice, cucumber, ginger, coconut oil, ice and protein powder in the blender. Blend on high speed until smooth, mix in the maple syrup and serve.

Fruit Salad-

You will need:

2 cups of spinach, fresh and chopped

½ an apple, sliced

5 strawberries, sliced

1 banana, sliced

1 orange, peeled and separated into pieces

1 tbsp Chia seeds

1 tbsp of your favorite peanut butter

2 tablespoons of fresh lemon juice

Begin by placing your spinach on the plate and top with your fruit, creating a visually pleasing salad, sprinkle the lemon juice over the salad followed by the Chia seeds and place the 1 tablespoon of peanut butter to the side to use for dipping.

Lunches

Vegetarian Chili-

You will need:

2 tbsp. Coconut oil

1 onion, chopped

2 bell peppers, red, seeded and chopped

1 butternut squash, about 1.5 pounds, peeled and chopped into cubes

4 cloves of garlic, minced

1 tbsp. Chili powder

½ tbsp. Chipotle pepper

1 tsp. Cumin

¼ tsp. Cinnamon

1 bay leaf

2 15 ounce cans of black beans

1 14 ounce can of diced tomatoes

2 cups of vegetable broth (about 14 ounces)

2 avocados, pits and peel removed, diced

Corn tortillas or corn tortilla chips

Salt to taste

Begin by placing a large stock pot (4-6 quarts) over medium heat, placing the coconut oil in the pot allowing it to begin to simmer. Once the oil has melted and begun to simmer, place the onion, butternut squash, and bell pepper into the pot, stirring until the onions begin to turn translucent.

Reduce the heat to low, adding in the chili powder, chipotle peppers, cinnamon, garlic, and cumin. Stir constantly for about 30 seconds, then adds in the bay leaf.

Next, you will add the can of diced tomatoes as well as the juice, black beans (rinsed) and the vegetable broth. Stir well then cover, cooking for about an hour. Make sure you stir this occasionally to ensure it does not stick to the bottom of the pan.

After the mixture has cooked for about 30 minutes, taste the mixture to determine you would like to add more chipotle peppers.

Your chili will be finished cooking when the squash is tender and you will notice that the liquid has been reduced slightly. Salt.

In order to make tortilla strips, you will slice your corn tortillas, this is easily done if you stack them. Each strip should be about ¼ of an inch wide and 2 inches in length. Drizzle olive oil in a medium skillet and heat it over medium heat. Place the sliced tortilla in the oil and sprinkle with salt. Cook until the strips turn golden brown and are crispy. You should stir them while they cook and the process will take up to 7 minutes.

After they have cooked, you can remove them from the oil and allow the oil to drain off of them on a plate covered with a paper towel.

To serve the chili you will place it in a bowl, top it with the tortilla strips and avocado. Sprinkle with cilantro to garnish.

Lentil Soup

You will need:

¼ cup EVOO (extra virgin olive oil)

1 onion, chopped

2 carrots, chopped

4 cloves of garlic, minced

2 tsp. Cumin

1 tsp. Curry powder

½ tsp. Thyme

28 ounces of diced tomatoes, drained

1 cup lentils, brown or green, rinsed and picked over

4 c. Vegetable broth

2 c. Water

1 tsp. Salt

Red pepper flakes

Black pepper

1 cup collard greens or kale, chopped, ribs removed

The juice of 1 lemon

Directions:

Begin by placing the EVOO in a large stock pot on the stove over medium heat. Once the oil has begun to simmer, you can add in the carrots and onions allowing to cook for about five minutes until the onions turn translucent. Make sure to stir often.

Next, you will add the cumin, thyme, curry powder and garlic, allowing to cook for about 30 seconds before pouring in the drained diced tomatoes. Allow to cook for about 2 minutes and then mix in the lentils, water and vegetable broth along with a pinch of red pepper flakes, and 1 teaspoon of salt. Season with black pepper and bring to a boil by raising the heat.

Once the mixture has reached a boil, reduce the heat again, partially cover and cook for about 30 minutes until the lentils are tender. Do not overcook if the lentils begin to lose their shape they have cooked for too long.

After the soup has cooked for about 30 minutes, remove two cups of the soup and place it in a blender, blending until smooth, then place the puree back into the soup pot, and add in the collard greens or Kale.

Allow to cook for about 5 more minutes, then remove from heat and add the lemon juice, stirring well, add salt and pepper to taste then serve.

Lentil and Chickpea Salad

You will need:

2 cups black beluga lentils

2 cloves of garlic, sliced in half lengthwise

2 tablespoons of coconut oil

For the dressing you will need:

The juice of 2 lemons

2 tbsp. EVOO

1 tsp. Dijon mustard

1 tsp. Honey

1 clove of garlic, minced

¼ tsp. Salt

Pepper to taste

For the salad, you will need:

1 can 14 ounces of chickpeas, drained and rinsed

Radishes, 1 large bunch, sliced thinly and then chopped

¼ cup of mint and dill mixed and chopped

Avocado, sliced

Feta for garnish

Directions:

You will begin by picking over the lentils, making sure that you remove any bits of debris and then rinsing them under cold water. Once you have picked over the lentils, place them in a medium-sized pot with the cloves of garlic, coconut oil and 4 cups of water.

Bring the mixture to a boil, then reduce the heat, allowing it to simmer gently until the lentils are tender which should take about 30 minutes.

After the lentils have drained, drain the mixture, discarding the garlic.

In order to make the dressing you will place all of the ingredients in a bowl and whisk well.

Finally, place the lentils, chopped radishes, herbs (mint and dill) into a large bowl add the dressing and toss well. Serve topped with avocado or feta.

Pasta Salad

You will need:

For the Pasta Salad, you will need:

½ a pound of your favorite whole grain pasta (penne, bow-tie, or rotini)

1 can of black beans (14 ounces) drained and rinsed well

10 ounces of cherry tomatoes, sliced thinly into rounds

1 fresh ear of corn, about ½ cup of corn kernels shucked

½ cup Feta or 1 avocado, diced

For the Pesto, you will need:

1 cup of parsley, fresh and packed lightly

1 cup of cilantro, fresh and packed lightly

1 jalapeno, seeds and membranes removed, chopped

The juice of one lemon

1 clove of garlic, chopped

½ teaspoon of salt

½ cup of green pumpkin seeds (slivered almonds work well too)

½ cup EVOO

Black pepper

Directions-

You will begin by cooking your pasta to al dente, following the directions on the package. Before you drain the pasta, you will need to take out one cup of the water that the pasta has cooked in and set to the side. Drain the pasta, then return it to the pot, it was cooked in and set it to the side.

Next, toast the green pumpkin seeds in a skillet over medium heat. Make sure that you stir frequently and cook until they begin to make a popping sound. They should also turn slightly golden around the edges. Remove from heat and set to the side to cool.

Now it is time to make the pesto. Begin by placing the lemon juice, garlic, salt, herbs and jalapeno in a food processor, follow with the pumpkin seeds. Pulse this mixture a few times and then begin drizzling the EVOO into the mixture, allowing the food processor to run the entire time, until it is well blended. You may need to stop and scrape the mixture down into the bowl as you are mixing it.

After you have created the pesto, you will pour it over the pasta, tossing the pasta until coated, (you do not have to use all of the pesto) Now you will take the cooking water that you sat to the side and add just a splash to the pasta, mix well.

Next, you will transfer the entire mixture to a serving bowl, add in the black beans, tomatoes and corn as well as the feta or avocado if you are using it. Combine well. Let sit for about 30 minutes, allowing the past to marinate then serve.

Kale and Apple Salad

You will need:

For the salad, you will need:

½ a cup of pecans, chopped

8 ounces of kale

5 radishes

½ a cup of dried cranberries

1 apple (Granny Smith works best)

2 ounces of goat cheese,

For the dressing, you will need:

3 Tbsp. EVOO

1 ½ tbsp. ACV (apple cider vinegar)

1 tbsp. Dijon mustard

1 ½ tsp. Honey

Salt and pepper to taste.

Directions:

You will begin by preheating your oven to 350 degrees and placing your pecans on a baking tray, toasting them until they are golden which will take about 5 minutes. During this time, you will toss them in order to ensure they are cooked evenly. When the pecans are finished, remove them from the oven and set them to the side allowing them to cool.

Next you will remove the tough ribs and stems from the kale and discard. Chop the kale into small pieces, then place it in a large bowl. Sprinkle a small bit of salt onto the Kale and then massage into the leaves by taking large handfuls and scrunching them in your hand. When the leaves have become dark in color and you can smell them, you are finished.

Take your radishes, chop off the root end, using the flat surface as a base, place them on your cutting board and cut into thin slices.

Chop pecans as well as the cranberries and place them along with the radishes into the large salad bowl with the kale. Next, you will chop the apple and add it to the salad as well, followed by crumbled goat cheese.

For the dressing, you will place all of the dressing ingredients in a small bowl and wish well, pour over salad and toss to ensure it is evenly coated. Serve immediately.

Veggie Hummus Wraps

You will need:

1 tortilla, or flavored wrap such as spinach

1/3 a cup of hummus, plain is fine, or flavored such as Spicy Roasted Red Pepper

2 slices of a cucumber, cut lengthwise

A handful of spinach

2 tomato slices

¼ avocado, sliced

Broccoli sprouts

Micro Greens

Basil leaves

Begin by spreading the hummus on the wrap. Choose one side, and leave about ½ an inch at the bottom of the wrap, but spread the hummus all the way to the sides of the wrap.

Next place the spinach, tomato slices, sprouts, basil, microgreens and cucumber onto the wrap and fold just as you would a burrito. Cut in half and serve.

Miso Soup

You will need:

5 cups of vegetable broth

1 oz. of shiitake mushrooms, dried

.5 pound of firm tofu, cut it into cubes that are about ¼ of an inch

1 sheet nori, cut this into squares about 1 inch in size

2 tsp ginger

2 cups broccoli florets (you should focus on getting small florets)

1 cup carrot, grated

4 tbsp. Miso

You will begin by pouring the vegetable broth into a large stock pot and bringing it to a boil. Once the broth has been brought to a boil, remove it from the heat, adding in the shiitake mushrooms. Then cover and let sit for about 20 minutes, allowing the mushrooms to soften.

After the mushrooms have softened, you will use a slotted spoon to remove the mushrooms from the broth, cut off the stems, discarding them and then cutting the cap of the mushrooms into thin slices. Set the mushrooms to the side.

Place the broth back on the stove, add in the nori, ginger and tofu, bring the mixture to a simmer and allow to cook for about three minutes.

Next you will place the mushrooms back into the pot along with the carrots and broccoli florets. Cover the soup and allow to cook for about 1 minute or until the broccoli becomes bright green in color. Place 1 cup of the broth from the soup into a small bowl and stir in the miso. Use a fork to stir the miso into the broth, stirring until the miso has completely dissolved.

Pour the mixture back into the pot and mix well to ensure the miso is mixed in completely. Serve.

Dinners-

Veggie Pizza-

You will need:

2 tsp. Dry yeast

1 c. Warm water

3 c. All- purpose flour

1 tbsp. Sugar

1 tbsp. Oregano, dried

1 tsp. Salt

1 egg

1 tbsp. EVOO

1 tbsp. Oregano, dried

1 garlic clove, chopped finely

1 tsp. Onion powder

1 tsp. Kosher salt

1 onion chopped finely

Black pepper

1.25 c. Mozzarella cheese, shredded

.5 c. Bell peppers, chopped, (green works best)

.5 cup of onion, chopped

Begin by placing the warm water in a bowl and sprinkling the yeast over the top of it. You need to make sure that the water is not hotter than 100 degrees. Let this stand for about 5 minutes, or until the yeast begins to form a foam.

Sift together the 1 tbsp. Oregano, 1 tsp. Salt and flour into a large bowl. Next, you will mix in the eggs and the EVOO into the flour mixture, followed by the yeast mixture. Once the dough has come together, you will knead it until it becomes smooth and elastic. This will take about 8 minutes.

Lightly oil a bowl large enough to place the dough in and then place the dough in it, coating the dough with the oil. Place the dough to the side and let rise for about 1 hour.

After the dough has risen, you will preheat your oven to 450 degrees and lightly grease a pizza pan.

Place a saucepan over medium heat, add in the diced tomatoes, tomato paste, one onion chopped finely, 1 tbsp. Oregano, garlic, 1 tsp. Salt, pepper and onion powder in the saucepan and cook until it thickens. This will take about 20 minutes.

Punch down on the dough, then place it on a floured surface. Divide the dough into two pieces that are equal in size using a knife. Now you will begin shaping the dough into balls and let rest for another 10 minutes.

After the dough has rested, you can shape the dough for your pizza according to the shape of your pizza pan. Place the dough on your pizza pan, then spoon the sauce over the dough. Sprinkle 1.25 cups of shredded mozzarella cheese on the pizza and top with bell peppers, onions and mushrooms. Top with another .25 cups of mozzarella cheese.

Bake for about 25 minutes or until the crust has become crisp and the cheese has melted.

Spinach Enchiladas

You will need:

1 tbsp. Butter

5 c. Green onions, chopped

1 garlic clove, minced

1 package of spinach (thawed, drained, squeezed and chopped)

1 c. Ricotta

½ c. Sour cream

2 c. Shredded Monterey Jack

10 corn tortillas

1 can of enchilada sauce (19 ounce)

Directions:

Begin by placing a saucepan on the stove over medium heat and melting the butter. After the butter has melted you can add the onion and the garlic cooking for a few minutes but not allowing to brown.

After you have cooked the garlic, stir in the spinach and allow to cook for about five minutes.

Remove the mixture from the heat, mix in the sour cream, 1 cup of Monterey Jack and ricotta. Next, you will heat, the tortilla shells in a skillet over medium heat. It should take about 15 seconds per shell.

Place ¼ of a cup of your spinach mixture each tortilla shell, roll the shell and place each one of them with the seam side down in a baking dish. Pour the enchilada sauce over the top of the enchiladas and sprinkle with one cup of Monterey Jack cheese. Bake the enchiladas for about 20 minutes or until the cheese is lightly brown at the edges and the sauce begins to bubble. Serve.

Quinoa and black beans

You will need:

1 tsp. Coconut oil

1 chopped onion

3 garlic cloves, chopped

¾ cup of quinoa

1 ½ c. Vegetable broth

1 tsp. Cumin

¼ tsp. Cayenne pepper

Salt and pepper

1 cup corn kernels, frozen

2 cans of black beans (15 ounce cans) drained and rinsed

½ cup of cilantro, fresh and chopped

Directions:

Begin by placing the oil in a saucepan over medium heat. Melt the oil, then add in the onions and garlic, cooking until they have begun to brown or about 10 minutes. Place the quinoa into the pan, then cover it with vegetable broth.

Add the cayenne pepper, salt, cumin, and pepper, bringing the mixture to a boil. Once the mixture has reached a boil, reduce heat and cover, allowing the quinoa to simmer until it is tender and has absorbed the broth. This will take about 20 minutes.

Mix the frozen corn into the quinoa and allow to cook for about five more minutes before adding in the black beans and cilantro. Serve hot.

Black Bean Veggie Burgers

You will need:

1 can of black beans (16 ounces) rinsed and drained

½ of a green bell pepper with the seeds removed, cut into 1-2 inch pieces

½ of an onion cut into wedges

3 garlic cloves, peeled

1 egg

1 tbsp. Chili powder

1 tsp. Hot sauce

½ c. Bread crumbs

Directions:

Begin by preheating your oven to 375 degrees, then lightly oil your baking sheet.

Next, place your black beans in a medium bowl and smash them with a fork until they become thick like paste. Place your bell pepper, onion and garlic into a food processor and pulse until smooth.

After you have blended the bell pepper, onion and garlic in the food processor, place the mixture in the bowl with the black beans and mix well.

In a separate bowl, mix the egg, cumin, chili sauce and chili powder together. Pour the egg mixture into the bean mixture and add in the bread crumbs.

Mix everything together until it holds together and becomes sticky. Divide the mixture into four parts and shape into patties.

Place the patties on the oiled baking sheet and bake for 10 minutes before flipping the burgers and baking for another 10 minutes.

Serve on a whole wheat bun with your favorite burger toppings.

Zucchini Grinders

You will need:

For the sauce:

1 tbsp. EVOO

2 garlic cloves, peeled and then chopped, coarsely

1 pinch of red pepper flakes

1 tbsp. Basil, fresh and chopped

1 tsp. Red wine vinegar

1 tsp. White sugar

1 can of diced tomatoes (14.5 ounce can)

Salt and pepper to taste

For the Grinders:

1 tbsp. Butter

2 zucchinis, cubed

1 pinch of red pepper flakes

Salt and pepper to taste

1.5 c. Mozzarella cheese

4 Italian sandwich rolls, 6 inches, split

Directions-

To begin making the marinara sauce you will need to place a saucepan on the stove over medium heat and place the oil inside of the pan. Once the oil has heated, add in the red pepper flakes, basil and garlic cooking for 2 minutes stirring the entire time.

Next, you will add the salt, pepper, salt, vinegar and sugar to the pan, followed by the diced tomatoes as well as the juices that are in the can. Mix well and simmer for 15 minutes. Remove the mixture from the stove and place in a food processor or blender, blending until smooth.

After you have made the marinara sauce, you will preheat your oven to 350 degrees. While the oven is preheating, place a skillet on the stove over medium heat and melt the butter in the skillet. Place your zucchini in the skillet and cook until it had become tender and begun to brown. Season with salt, pepper and red pepper flakes if desired.

After the zucchini has cooked, place a large amount into each roll, cover with ¼ cup of the sauce and top with mozzarella cheese. After you have filled each roll, you will close it, and wrap in foil.

Bake the rolls for 15 minutes or until the rolls are soft and the cheese has melted.

Eggplant Sandwiches

You will need:

8 eggplant slices that are about ½ an inch think

2 tsp. EVOO divided

1 red bell pepper, large

4 ciabatta bread slices

2 tbsp. Pesto

1 c. Baby arugula

1/8 tsp black pepper

2 ounces (1/4 c.) Goat cheese, soft

Directions:

Begin by preheating the broiler. Place the eggplant slices on a baking sheet lined with foil, in a single layer. Brush each side of the eggplant with one teaspoon of the EVOO. Cut your bell peppers in half lengthwise and then discard the seeds. Place cut-side down on the baking sheet and use the palm of your hand to flatten out the bell pepper halves.

Broil the eggplant and bell peppers for 4 minutes, turn the eggplant over, leaving the bell pepper as is and broil for 4 more minutes. Remove the eggplant from the pan and set to the side. Allow the bell pepper to broil for 7 more minutes. The bell peppers should be blackened when they are done.

Place the peppers in a zip-lock bag and seal the bag, allowing the peppers to sit for 15 minutes before peeling them and discarding the skin.

Place the ciabatta bread on a baking sheet and broil for 2 minutes until they are lightly brown, turning them once as they broil.

On each 2 of the slices of bread you will spread 1 tbsp. of pesto. Place 2 eggplant slices on top of the

2 slices of bread with pesto, followed by 1 of the bell pepper halves and two more slices of eggplant.

In a small bowl, mix the arugula, 1 tsp. EVOO and black pepper, then divide the mixture between the sandwiches. Finally, spread 2 tbsp. of the soft goat cheese over the remaining 2 slices of bread and place them on the top of the sandwich, cheese side down. Serve.

Baked Ziti

You will need:

4 ounces of uncooked, whole wheat ziti

1 tbsp. EVOO

2 cups yellow squash, chopped

1 cup zucchini, chopped

½ cup onion, chopped

2 cups of tomato, chopped

2 cloves of garlic, minced

4 ounces, mozzarella cheese, shredded, divided

2 tbsp. Basil, fresh and chopped

2 tsp. Oregano, fresh and chopped

¾ tsp. Salt, divided

1/8 tsp. Crushed red pepper

2 ounces or ¼ cup of ricotta

1 egg, beaten lightly

Nonstick cooking spray

Begin by cooking your pasta according to the directions on the package, but leave out the salt and the fat. After you have cooked the pasta, preheat your oven to 400 degrees.

Place a large skillet on the stove over medium to high heat and place EVOO in the pan. After the oil has heated up, add in the zucchini, onions and squash allowing to saute for about five minutes.

Next, you will add the garlic and tomato, sautéing for an additional three minutes, then removing from the heat. Stir the pasta into the vegetable mix as well as ½ a cup of mozzarella, basil, oregano, salt and pepper.

In a separate bowl, mix the ricotta, egg and remaining salt, then add the pasta mixing well. Place the pasta mixture into an 8-inch square baking pan that has been coated with nonstick cooking spray and sprinkle with the rest of the mozzarella cheese. Bake for 15 minutes or until the cheese begins to brown around the edge.

Chapter 5- Tips to Maximize the Use of Vegetarian Diets for Weight Loss

Although a vegetarian diet is extremely healthy and chances are you are going to lose weight, especially if you follow what you have learned in this book, if you do not follow the diet properly, you are not going to lose weight. Remember, I talked about overweight vegetarians earlier in this book? For that reason, I want to give you a few tips that you can use to ensure your success at losing weight while on a vegetarian diet.

1. **What foods to avoid:**

The first thing that I want to tell you is that you need to avoid processed foods as much as possible. While it may be okay for you to eat an entire cake, according to a vegetarian diet, it is not okay if you want to lose weight. Processed foods are simply foods that are made in a lab, they are not real food, and they are nothing more than empty calories. For that reason, you want to avoid, baked goods, white bread and flours, refined sugars, soda, full-fat dairy products, and candy. Basically, if the food has been highly processed, you need to avoid it if you want to lose weight.

2. When you should eat.

It is important for you to know when you should eat. You never want to get too hungry when you are on any type of diet. In fact, you should eat three meals per day and two snacks in between each meal while staying within your daily caloric needs. If you allow yourself to become too hungry, you will only slow your metabolic rate, therefore slowing the rate that you lose weight.

3. Oil is important.

While you will need to use oil to make specific meals you want to get away from liquid oils if possible. Coconut oil is a great choice to cook with and will provide you with many health benefits, but you can also use cooking sprays. EVOO cooking sprays can be used instead of oil, ensuring that you are not adding a lot of fat to your foods that you are eating, therefore, ensuring that you are losing weight. However, it is not recommended that you eliminate all fats from your diet. I do suggest getting at least 2 tablespoons of coconut oil into your diet each day because your body simply will not burn fat without getting enough fat. Coconut oil is the right kind of fat for your body because it is the only fat that has been proven to not turn into fat.

4. Snacks.

Snacks are very important, but you do not want them to be packed full of calories. Instead, you want them to be packed full of fiber. Fruits and vegetables are great snacks, but you need to be careful when it comes to the types of fruits that you snack on as well as the amount of fruit that you are eating. Fruits are full of sugar, just like refined sugar, if you eat too much of this sugar, it is going to turn into fat, even though it is natural sugar. Fruits such as bananas are loaded with sugar and should be eaten in limited quantities. While you do not want to eliminate bananas from your diet completely, you do want to watch the amount that you eat.

5. Exercise is Important

One thing that I have not covered in this book was exercise so I want to take a few moments to talk about it. Exercise is necessary for you to lose weight. We live in a world today where we are so busy, we barely have time to add anything to our days, but exercise is a must if we want to lose weight and become healthy. Exercise is going to build muscle; muscle is going to burn more calories while making you look even better. If you are just starting out, adding exercise into your daily routine may seem impossible, and it is the reason that so many people fail when they are dieting. Most people jump right in, thinking that they are going to exercise for an hour a day, seven days a week, and when they find that this is all but impossible for beginners, they give up.

Instead of setting yourself up for failure by setting outrageous goals, set reachable goals. If you can only exercise for 5 minutes at a time, set that as your goal. Five minutes a day, seven days per week. Then each week, add another five minutes until you are exercising for 60 minutes a day with no problems.

You need to focus on aerobic exercise to begin with, later you can add strength training and stretching exercises such as yoga if desired.

6. Water is Important as Well.

If you want to be successful at losing weight, no matter what diet you are using, you need to make sure that you are drinking a lot of water. It is recommended that you drink at least 8, 8 ounce glasses of water per day or 64 ounces, however if you are dehydrated, you need to make sure you are drinking more. If you are not getting enough water, your body is not going to burn calories like it would if you were hydrated. In other words, not drinking water can literally slow down your metabolism. Not only can it slow down your metabolism, but it can slow you down as well. You for the coffee when you wake up each morning, try a big glass of water with a spritz of lemon juice and watch your energy levels skyrocket.

7. Stay away from the scale.

The truth is that the scale is going to lie to you. You can lose inches on your body while gaining weight. Of course, this is going to even out over time, but what is happening is that you are losing fat while gaining muscle. Since the muscle takes up much less space that the fat, you will notice a change in the way your clothes fit you, but you may not notice a change in the number on the scale. Weighing once per week is fine, but the rest of the time, stay away from the scale.

8. Be Prepared.

If you are going from a diet full of processed foods and meats to a vegetarian diet, you need to be prepared for what is going to happen specifically cravings. When you eliminate processed foods from your diet, you are going to crave those refined sugars, just like a drug addict craves their drug. You see, sugar has the same effect on your brain, and you will not feel 100 percent for the first few days. Do not give into these cravings because each time you give into them; you extend the time it takes your body to stop craving them. The same goes for meat products. Simply knowing that this is going to happen is going to help prepare you for it. Have a plan, know what are you going to do to take your mind off of the cravings.

Conclusion

We as humans were made to eat food that comes from the Earth. We were not made to eat chemicals that are formed into what we call food today. When you start eating a vegetarian diet, as long as you do not become a junk food vegetarian, you are going to begin seeing all of that extra weight fall right off of your body.

I am not going to lie and tell you that a vegetarian diet is easy in the beginning, you have to learn how to cook new foods, and there are going to be times when you simply cannot stand the way vegetables taste. However, it does get easier with time, and as long as you eat a variety of foods and meals, you will not have problems sticking to the diet.

In fact, when you begin feeling better than you have ever felt before, having more energy than you have ever had before and when you begin seeing the weight literally melt off, you will become even more motivated to stick to your vegetarian diet.

I hope that in this book you have found the information that you need to help you get started on your weight loss journey by a vegetarian diet. Your next step is to begin experimenting with foods, learning some new favorite recipes and get ready to go shopping for some new, smaller clothes.

Finally, do not become discouraged, if you reach a point in your diet where you become stuck and don't feel as if you are making progress, don't give up. Keep pushing and you will push through that wall. Everyone hits these points where it seems that they are stuck and are not seeing the results they want to see, and this is when many people give up on their diet but don't let that stop you. Take an honest look at what you have been eating and how much have been exercising, jump back on the fast track to weight loss and don't let the wall stop you.

Lose Weight: On a Healthy Vegetarian Diet

Copyright ©2016 by CHARLES BENSON